THE SOUTH BEACH DIET

*The South Beach Diet Guide for Beginners
with Complete Meal Plan & Delicious
Recipes to Get Healthy and Lose Weight Fast*

Table of Contents

Introduction 1

Free Bonus Book...3

Chapter 1 All About The South Beach Diet........................5

The Three Phases of the South Beach Diet............................ 8

Chapter 2 Phase 1 Sample Meal Plan For 14 Days 13

Day 1.. 13

Day 2.. 19

Day 3..25

Day 4.. 30

Day 5..37

Day 6..43

Day 7 51

Day 8..58

Day 9..63

Day 10 69

Day 11..76

Day 12 81

Day 13 88

Day 14 95

Chapter 3 Phases 2 And 3 Recipes 101

Breakfast Recipes *101*

Lunch Recipes *115*

Dinner *129*

Snacks/Desserts/Beverages *139*

Conclusion 155

Thank You! 156

INTRODUCTION

I want to thank you and congratulate you for purchasing the book, *"South Beach Diet: The South Beach Diet Guide for Beginners with Complete Meal Plan & Delicious Recipes to Get Healthy and Lose Weight Fast"*

This book contains proven steps and strategies on how to achieve your desired weight through the help of the South Beach Diet.

The South Beach Diet is not like the other low-carb diets that you know as you don't have to completely eliminate or minimize your consumption of carbohydrates. This diet is grounded on the principle that one has to remove bad carbohydrates and bad fats into their diet in order to lose weight effectively.

In this book, you will learn the principles of the South Beach Diet, how it works, the food that you are allowed to eat and avoid, and a complete meal plan and recipes for breakfast, lunch, dinner, and snacks. The game plan here is to decrease the consumption of bad carbs, which in turn could decrease weight at a rapid pace, metabolize carbs properly, and insulin resistance starts to clear up on its own.

The South Beach diet is very successful and is favored by many people because you can still eat your favorite food provided that you avoid the bad carbs and fats. If you want to get to know more about this diet and the many recipes that you can make in order to follow this program, read on the pages that follow.

Thanks again for purchasing this book. I hope you enjoy it!

FREE BONUS BOOK

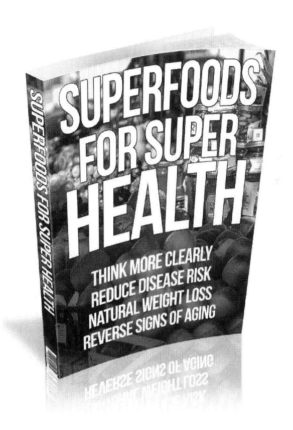

As a Thank You for purchasing this book, I would like to offer you another book as a special bonus! It is called "Super Foods For Super Health".

This comprehensive book is for those who are interested in:

- Learning more about super foods that you can easily get your hands on today.
- How to incorporate those super foods into your everyday meals.
- Nutritional benefits for each super foods
- How to improve your overall health
- How to lose weight naturally
- How to reduce disease risk
- How to reverse signs of aging
- Think more clearly
- Improving your focus
- And much more..

So if you are interested in learning more about any of the above, just go to http://bit.ly/superfoods-gift and grab your free bonus book!

Chapter 1
All about the South Beach Diet

The South Beach diet was initially designed by Dr. Agatston to help improve the condition of his patients suffering from chronic heart diseases. The foods included in this diet are heart-friendly. Through weeks and months of adhering to said diet, he was surprised how his patients have made a significant improvement with regards to their overall health.

When Dr. Agatston published his first book, many health enthusiasts tried the diet to see if it is effective for weight loss. And, they were not disappointed as the diet program has proven that weight loss is indeed achievable.

According to studies, fats are good for one's health. In fact, you do not have to avoid all fats in your diet. But, make sure they are good fats.

Good fats are classified into 2 types: the monounsaturated fats and the polyunsaturated fats. Monounsaturated fats are usually found in food such as avocados, oatmeal, peanuts, cashews, olive oil, sesame oil, macadamia nuts, and peanut butter. On the other hand, Polyunsaturated fats are found in tuna, salmon, sardines, whole grain wheat, almonds, flax seeds, soybeans, and seaweeds. These are known as Omega- 3 fatty acids and are considered good for the heart. This type of fat is also good at treating other illnesses such as diabetes, arthritis, asthma, depression, and heart diseases.

Now where are the bad fats? Saturated fats are mostly found in red meats, full fat milk, and butter. Trans fats also known as "lethal fats" are also bad for one's health. These include junk food, donuts, cakes, cookies, and other sweet treats. Trans fats can cause obesity, bloating, and can also affect the proper functioning of your nervous system.

The South Beach diet also promotes the consumption of good carbohydrates. Some of the good carbs include wheat bread, vegetables, whole grain rice, and legumes. Bad carbohydrates, on the other hand, include foods that contain refined starches. Some examples include pasta, white rice, white bread, crackers, and biscuits.

The Principle of the South Beach is very simple - remove the bad carbs and bad fats from your daily diet and you will reap great results. After weeks and months of religiously following this diet, you will see a healthier, fitter, and leaner you.

The Three Phases of the South Beach Diet

South Beach Diet Phase 1

The first phase lasts for 14 days. You are expected to lose weight somewhere between 8 – 13 pounds in the first 2 weeks of following said diet. During this phase, your cravings should be minimized and your blood sugar levels stabilized.

What are the foods allowed during this stage?

- Fruits such as: avocado, lemon juice, lime juice
- Vegetables such as: okra, squash, spinach, sprouts, cauliflower, radish, chickpeas, broccoli, eggplant, zucchini, cabbage, rhubarb, garbanzo, bok choy, lettuce, tomato, cucumber, olives, snow peas
- Beef cuts such as: tenderloin, ground beef, sirloin, top loin, and top round.
- Pork cuts such as: tenderloin, ham (broiled), pork loin, bacon, Fat free luncheon meat
- Lamb cuts such as : loins and chops
- Veal
- Skinless turkey and chicken breast

- Fish
- Shellfish
- Mushrooms
- Soy products such as: tofu, soy beans, soy nuts, soy milk, Fat free
- Protein food such as: eggs, milk (fat free), low fat cheese or Fat free (mozzarella, cheddar, Parmesan, feta, ricotta, cottage cheese, and cream cheese)
- Spreads such as: Peanut butter, guacamole, mayonnaise (low fat)
- Sauces and Salsa such as: Worcestershire Sauce, salad dressing (low fat), hot sauce
- Broth
- Condiments such as: cayenne pepper, cocoa powder, sugar substitutes, chocolate powder (no sugar added)
- Others: gelatin, sugar free

Food to Avoid:
- Fatty meat
- Butter
- coconut oil
- Fatty poultry

- Whole milk
- Grains
- refined sugar
- Honey
- maple syrup
- agave nectar
- All fruits and fruit juice especially those that are high in sugar
- Vegetables such as: yams, beets, carrots, white potatoes, corn, turnips, peas, and winter squash
- Alcohol

South Beach Diet Phase 2

During this phase, a south beach dieter may continue to consume the foods that are not allowed during Phase 1. It is during this phase when you can add up on your servings, say 3 servings of fruits and starchy veggies, brown rice, wheat bread, and quinoa. You may also have one serving of dark chocolate or wine.

However, you should take note that you still need to avoid eating instant oatmeal, white rice, cornflakes, bagels, and white pasta. You should also avoid fruits with high sugar content such as mangoes, pineapples, and dates. The very concept of Phase 2 is to slowly reintroduce yourself to high fiber, low glycemic carbohydrates.

The secret is that you eat fewer food that usually trigger cravings. Some of the food that you took out from Phase 1 can be added back to your diet only that you do so less often. So let's say you wanted bread for breakfast, you can have it but not every day.

As you go through this phase, your weight loss will be reduced not drastically, but it will be consistent. You can expect to lose 2 pounds in a week. While this is definitely lower from that of Phase 1, still, losing weight slowly is healthier and you will be able to keep it off for long.

South Beach Diet Phase 3

This phase will only start once you have achieved your desired weight. After you have gone through Phases 1 and 2, it would be easier to stay in this phase for the rest of your life. You will notice that your body is now trained to make healthy food choices. This phase feels like normal eating once again only that you are more aware of the kind of food to consume and are good for your health. Should you feel that you are getting a little off track during this phase, just try to modify the amount and the kind of food that you are eating.

In a Nutshell

As you lose weight and get healthier through the South Beach Diet, your cardiovascular system will improve and your blood chemistry will change. So even if your goal is to lose weight through the South Beach Diet, in the end, you will notice that you have achieved so much more!

Chapter 2
Phase 1 Sample Meal Plan for 14 Days

This Chapter includes recipes for breakfast, lunch, dinner, and snacks for 14 days

Day 1

Breakfast - Asparagus and Broccoli Frittata

Ingredients:

- 6 thick-stemmed asparagus
- 2 eggs, whisked until frothy
- 1 broccoli head, sliced into bite-sized florets
- 1 garlic clove, minced
- 1 ripe tomato, minced
- 1 onion, minced
- 1 Tbsp. olive oil
- Pinch of sea salt, add more if needed
- Pinch of black pepper, to taste

Optional

- 1 Tbsp. parsley, minced

Directions:

1. Preheat the oven to 375°F.

2. Pour olive oil into the skillet. Sauté onion and garlic for 3 minutes or until limp and aromatic. Add in tomato. Cook for 3 minutes or until the tomatoes soften.

3. Stir in broccoli florets. Season with salt and pepper. Cook for another 3 minutes. Turn off the heat.

4. Lightly grease a round deep pie dish with olive oil. Pour eggs and broccoli. Whisk well to combine.

5. Layer asparagus slivers on top. Cover with aluminum foil. Bake for 45 minutes.

6. Remove from oven and let sit for 5 minutes. Slice frittata into equal slices. Garnish with parsley. Serve.

Lunch - Stir-Fried Shrimps and Snow Peas

Ingredients:
- 1 tsp. olive oil
- 1 onion, minced
- 1 garlic clove, minced
- ½ lb. frozen shrimps, thawed
- 2 lbs. snow peas
- ¼ cup cashew nuts, garlic-roasted, store-bought
- Pinch of sea salt, add more if needed
- Pinch of black pepper, to taste

Directions:
1. Pour olive oil into a non-stick skillet. Sauté onion and garlic for 3 minutes or until limp and fragrant.
2. Add in shrimps, snow peas, and cashew nuts. Season with salt and pepper. Stir fry mixture for 3 minutes or until snow peas turn a shade brighter. Turn off the heat.
3. To serve, spoon equal portions into plates.

Snacks/Desserts/Beverages

Artichoke Hearts

Ingredients:
- olive oil, for shallow frying
- 1 pound artichoke hearts, quartered
- 1 cup almond flour, finely milled
- 2 eggs, whisked
- 1 cup almond meal
- Pinch of sea salt, add more if needed
- Pinch of white pepper, to taste
- ½ lemon, sliced into wedges

Directions:
1. Pour olive oil into a non-stick skillet. Season artichoke hearts with salt and pepper. Dredge in this order: almond flour, eggs, and almond meal.
2. Slide breaded artichokes into the hot pan. Fry until golden and crisp. Transfer to a plate. Drain on paper towels.
3. To serve, squeeze in lime juice over vegetables.

Dinner

Tuna Wraps with Olive Mayo

Ingredients:

For the Mayo

- ⅛ cup mayonnaise
- ½ tsp. Dijon mustard
- 1 garlic clove, grated
- 1 Tbsp. capers in brine, drained lightly, minced
- 1 black Kalamata olives in brine, minced
- 1 Tbsp. lemon juice
- ½ tsp. lemon zest, grated
- 1/16 tsp. black pepper

For the Tuna

- 2 pieces tuna fillet, sliced into 2-inch long thick slivers
- Pinch of sea salt, add more if needed
- ¼ cup corn flour

For the Vegetable fillings

- 1 cup arugula
- ¼ cup cucumbers, diced
- 2 Tbsp. cilantro, minced

- 4 lettuce leaves
- Oil for spraying

Directions:

1. Preheat the oven to 400°F.
2. For the mayo, put together mayonnaise, Dijon mustard, garlic clove, capers in brine, Kalamata olives, lemon juice, lemon zest, and black pepper. Mix well. Set aside until ready to use.
3. Meanwhile, season tuna fillets with salt. Place in a colander to drain for 15 minutes.
4. Dredge tuna fillets in corn flour. Transfer fillets to a baking dish lined with parchment paper. Spray with oil.
5. Place in an Air Fryer basket. Cook for 7 minutes or until fish is golden brown. Remove from basket.
6. To serve, spread mayo on lettuce leaves. Put desired amount of arugula, cucumbers, and cilantro. Top off with tuna.
7. Roll lettuce. Serve immediately.

Day 2

Breakfast - Mexican Omelet

Ingredients:
- 1 cup canned pinto beans
- ½ lime, freshly squeezed
- Olive oil, for spraying
- 3 whole eggs
- 4 egg whites
- ½ cup of guacamole
- ½ cup of salsa

Directions:
1. Put pinto beans into a food processor. Pour lime juice. Pulse until the mixture is similar to that of a refried beans.
2. Meanwhile, in a nonstick skillet, heat the olive oil cooking spray.
3. Whisk the whole eggs and egg whites. Divide the egg mixture into equal portions. Pour onto the pan.
4. Cook until the egg is set. Spoon just the right amount of bean mixture down the center of the omelet. Fold over a third of the omelet.

5. Transfer to a serving dish. Put guacamole and salsa on top. Serve.

Lunch - Lentils in Vegetable Soup

Ingredients:
- 1 tbsp. olive oil
- 4 leeks, minced
- 1 can whole tomatoes
- 6 cups vegetable stock
- 2 cups brown lentils
- 1 can button mushrooms
- 1 bunch kale, sliced into thick strips
- 1 pinch fresh thyme, chopped
- Pinch of sea salt, add more if needed
- Pinch of white pepper, to taste

Directions:
1. Heat the olive oil into the Dutch oven. Sauté leeks for 3 minutes or until tender.
2. Pour canned tomatoes. Cook or 3 minutes whilst stirring often so the tomatoes will break up.
3. Pour vegetable stock, brown lentils, button mushrooms, kale, and thyme. Season with salt and pepper. Bring mixture to a boil.
4. Once boiling, reduce the heat. Let it simmer for 20 minutes or until lentils are tender.

5. Adjust seasoning if needed. Serve.

Dinner – Sweet Potato and Broccoli Soup

Ingredients:

- 1 sweet onion, minced
- 4 garlic cloves, grated
- 1 sweet potato, diced
- ½ cup cashew nuts, raw
- 2 lbs. fresh broccoli, roughly chopped
- 4 cups vegetable broth, low-sodium
- Dash of cayenne powder
- Pinch of sea salt, add more if needed
- Pinch of white pepper, to taste

Directions:

1. Put onion, garlic, sweet potato, cashew nuts, broccoli, vegetable broth and cayenne powder into a large saucepan. Bring to boil.
2. Once boiling, reduce the heat and let it simmer for 20 minutes. Secure lid. Simmer soup for 20 minutes.
3. Turn off heat. Transfer soup to an immersion blender. Adjust taste if needed.
4. Ladle soup into bowls. Serve warm.

Black Tea with Blackberries and Cinnamon

Ingredients:

- 4 cups water
- 1 lb. blackberries, reserve some for garnish
- 4 teabags black tea
- 1 2-inch long cinnamon stick

Directions:

1. Pour water in a pitcher. Add in blackberries, black tea, and cinnamon stick. Mix well. Place inside the fridge for 4 hours.
2. Discard cinnamon stick and teabags.
3. Pour tea with the remaining blackberries. Serve chilled.

Day 3

Breakfast - Bake Avocado

Ingredients:
- 2 eggs
- 1 ripe avocado, halved
- Pinch of sea salt, add more if needed
- Pinch of white pepper, to taste
- Dash of Spanish paprika
- Dash of dried pepper flakes
- 1 Tbsp. fresh chives, minced

Directions:
1. Preheat the oven to 425°F. Line a baking dish with parchment paper.
2. Layer avocado halves, cut-side up in baking dish. Crack in one egg into avocado cavities.
3. Place inside the oven and bake for 15 minutes or until the eggs are set. Remove from the oven.
4. Slide avocado halves into plates. Season with salt pepper, pepper, flakes, and paprika. Garnish with fresh chives. Serve.

Lunch - Minute Egg Salad Roll

Ingredients:

- 1 apple, diced
- 12 pcs. quail eggs, hardboiled, quartered
- ¼ tsp. lemon juice, freshly squeezed
- 1½ Tbsp. mayonnaise
- Pinch of sea salt, add more if needed
- Pinch of white pepper, to taste
- 6 iceberg lettuce leaves

Directions:

1. In a bowl, put together apple, quail eggs, lemon juice, and mayonnaise. Toss well to combine. Season well with salt and pepper.
2. Place just the right amount of the salad into folds of lettuce leaves. Serve.

Dinner - Smoked Salmon on Cucumber Disks

Ingredients:
- 1 large cucumber, sliced into thick medallions

For the salad
- ½ cup arugula leaves, julienned
- 1 tsp. dill fronds, minced
- ⅛ cup fresh chives, minced, reserve some for garnish
- 1 lime, sliced
- 2 Tbsp. extra virgin olive oil
- Pinch of sea salt, add more if needed
- Pinch of white pepper, to taste
- 10 oz. smoked salmon, sliced thinly

Directions:
1. Place cucumber slices on a tray lined with parchment paper. Place inside the fridge to chill for 1 hour or until ready to use.
2. Put together arugula leaves, dill fonds, chives, lime, and olive oil into the salad bowl. Mix well. Season with salt and pepper.

3. Spoon equal amounts on top of cucumber disks. Put salmon slices on top. Garnish with chives. Serve.

Kale Crisps

Ingredients:
- 1 lb. kale leaves, torn
- coconut oil, melted, for drizzling
- Pinch of sea salt, add more if needed

Directions:
1. Preheat the oven to 300°F. Line a baking sheet with parchment paper.
2. In a bowl, put together kale leaves and coconut oil. Toss well.
3. Spread kale leaves on a baking sheet. Season with salt. Drizzle in more coconut oil.
4. Place inside the oven and bake for 15 minutes. Let cool before serving.

Day 4

Breakfast - Mushroom and Egg

Ingredients:

- 1 cap Portobello mushroom, stem removed
- Pinch of sea salt, add more if needed
- Pinch of pepper, to taste
- 2 tbsp. olive oil, divided
- 1 egg
- ⅛ avocado, thinly sliced
- 2 egg whites

Directions:

1. Preheat the broiler. Line a baking sheet with tin foil.
2. Brush the mushroom cap with olive oil. Place the mushroom cap on the baking sheet.
3. Put in the broiler. Broil for 5 minutes. Cook the other side of the mushroom for another 5 minutes.
4. Meanwhile, heat the remaining olive oil in a pan.

5. Whisk egg whites and egg together. Pour eggs into the pan. Cook until eggs set. Remove from heat.
6. Slide scrambled eggs in the mushroom cap. Put avocado slices on top. Season with salt and pepper Serve.

Lunch - Fish and Shrimp Curry Soup

Ingredients:
- 1 Tbsp. olive oil
- 2 shallots, minced
- 2 garlic cloves, minced
- 1 ginger, crushed
- 2 cups fish stock, unsalted
- 1 red bell pepper, cubed
- 1 bird's eye chili, halved lengthwise
- 1 banana chili, halved lengthwise
- ½ Tbsp. curry powder
- 1 Tbsp. garam masala
- ¼ tsp. Spanish paprika
- Pinch of sea salt, add more if needed
- Pinch of black pepper, to taste
- 1 can coconut cream, divided
- 1 lb. white fish of choice, cubed
- 1 lb. shrimps
- 1 Tbsp. parsley, minced

Directions:
1. Pour olive oil into a Dutch oven. Saute shallots, garlic, and for 3 minutes or until limp and aromatic.

2. Pour fish stock, red bell pepper, bird's eye chili, banana chili, curry powder, garam masala, Spanish paprika, salt, pepper, and half the coconut cream into the Dutch oven. Cover the lid and bring mixture to a boil.

3. Add in white fish and shrimps. Stir. Cook for another 7 minutes or until the fish starts to flake. Turn off the heat. Pour remaining coconut cream.

4. To serve, ladle equal portions into bowls. Garnish with parsley.

Dinner - Whole Chicken

Ingredients:
- 1 whole chicken
- Pinch of sea salt, add more if needed
- Pinch of white pepper, to taste
- 2 sprigs fresh rosemary, whole
- 2 sprigs fresh oregano, whole
- 2 sprigs fresh thyme, whole

For the chicken
- 4 garlic cloves
- 1 lemon, quartered
- olive oil for greasing/drizzling

Directions:
1. Preheat the oven to 350°F. Line a roasting tin with aluminum foil. Grease with olive oil.
2. Season chicken with salt and pepper. Place on a roasting tin. Tie rosemary, oregano, and thyme together using a kitchen twine. Stuff with lemon into the chicken cavity.
3. Squeeze lemon wedges on top of the chicken. Put garlic heads around the chicken. Drizzle in olive oil.

4. Cover with aluminum foil. Place roasting tin at the lowermost part of the oven. Cook for 1 hour.

5. Remove the aluminum foil. Continue roasting for 30 minutes. Remove for the oven and let sit for 10 minutes.

6. Discard garlic heads, herbs, and lemon wedge.

7. To assemble, carve roasted chicken into pieces. Transfer on a serving plate. Serve.

Cauliflower Pops

Ingredients:

- 1 head cauliflower, sliced into bite-sized pieces
- 1 Tbsp. olive oil
- Pinch of sea salt, add more if needed

Directions:

1. Preheat the oven to 350°F. Line a baking sheet with parchment paper
2. Drizzle in olive over the cauliflower. Bake for 20 minutes or until cauliflower turns golden brown.
3. Remove from the oven. Season with salt. Serve.

Day 5

Breakfast - Baked Tomato, Eggs, and Chicken

Ingredients:
- ½ tbsp. olive oil
- 2 garlic cloves, chopped
- 1 can tomatoes, chopped, reserve juices
- Handful of basil leaves, shredded
- 2 eggs
- ¼ cup chicken strips

Directions:
1. Preheat the oven to 350 degrees F.
2. Pour olive oil into the skillet. Once hot, saute garlic and chopped tomatoes. Pour tomato juices.
3. Secure the lid and allow mixture to simmer for 10 minutes. Add in basil.
4. Meanwhile, place tomatoes and chicken strips in a baking dish. Crack the eggs. Season with salt and pepper.
5. Place baking dish inside the microwave oven. Heat for 10 minutes. Serve.

Lunch – Spicy Tomato and Cucumber Salad

Ingredients:

For the Dressing
- 1 Tbsp. apple cider vinegar
- 1 Tbsp. balsamic vinegar
- ½ cup basil leaves, julienned
- 1 Tbsp. lemon juice, freshly squeezed
- 1 Tbsp. extra virgin olive oil
- Pinch of sea salt, add more if needed
- Pinch of black pepper, to taste
- 1 cup, cos lettuce, torn
- 2 cucumbers, sliced thinly
- 1 head escarole, torn
- 5 cherry tomatoes, quartered
- 1 bird's eye chili, minced
- ½ cup black olives in oil, drained

Directions:
1. Whisk apple cider vinegar, balsamic vinegar, basil leaves, lemon juice, olive oil, salt, and pepper in a bowl. Continue stirring until the salt dissolves. Adjust taste if needed.

2. Meanwhile, put together lettuce, cucumbers, escarole, tomatoes, bird's eye chili, and black olives in a salad bowl. Drizzle in dressing. Toss well to combine.

3. To serve, put equal amounts of salad in a bowl. Serve.

Dinner - Steamed Crab Legs with Garlic-Lemon Butter

Ingredients:
- water for steaming

For Crab legs
- 4 lbs. King crab legs, frozen or fresh, halved
- 1 ginger, peeled, crushed
- 4 garlic cloves, peeled
- Pinch of sea salt, add more if needed
- 1 Tbsp. heaping Spanish paprika

For the Dip
- Drop of organic honey
- 1 cup of coconut vinegar
- Pinch of sea salt
- Pinch of black pepper, to taste

Directions:
1. Fill the steamer with water about ¾ full. Bring to a boil.
2. Wrap the crab legs, ginger, and garlic with aluminum foil. Season with Spanish paprika and salt before covering.

3. Place in a steaming basket and cook for 1 hour.
4. Meanwhile, put together honey, vinegar, salt, and pepper in a bowl. Mix until all ingredients are well combined. Set aside.
5. Take out from the steaming basket and allow to cool before discarding ginger and garlic.
6. Crack crab legs and place into bowls. Serve with the dip on the side.

Snacks/Desserts/Beverages

Zucchini Chips

Ingredients:

- 4 zucchini, thinly sliced
- 2 tbsp. apple cider vinegar
- 2 tbsp. olive oil
- Pinch of sea salt, add more if needed
- ¼ tsp. ground black pepper

Directions:

1. Preheat the oven to 225 degrees F. Put parchment paper onto the baking dish.
2. Put together apple cider vinegar, olive oil, salt, and pepper in a small mixing bowl. Add in sliced zucchini. Mix well until ingredients are well coated.
3. Layer zucchini in the prepared baking dish. Bake for 2 hours.
4. Remove from the oven and let cool for few minutes. Serve.

Day 6

Breakfast – Black Bean Omelet

Ingredients:
- 1 can black beans, drained
- 1 lime, freshly squeezed
- Hot sauce
- 4 eggs
- Pinch of salt, add more if needed
- Pinch of pepper, to taste
- 4 egg whites
- 4 tablespoons salsa, store bought
- ½ avocado, sliced

Directions:
1. Using a food processor, put black beans, lime juice, and hot sauce together. Process and pulse until all ingredients are ell incorporated.
2. Meanwhile, lightly coat a pan with oil. Whisk one egg and one egg white together in a bowl. Season with salt and pepper. Pour into the pan.

3. When the eggs are just set, put just the right amount of the black bean mixture in the center. Fold the omelet over. Slide in a serving plate.

4. Place ¼ of the salsa and avocado slices on top. Repeat with the remaining eggs. Serve.

Lunch – Chili Pinto Beans with Avocado

Ingredients:
- 1 tbsp. olive oil
- 2 cloves garlic, minced
- 1 onion, minced
- ½ lb cremini mushrooms, diced
- 1 zucchini, diced
- 1 red bell pepper, diced
- 1 can tomatoes
- 1 can pinto beans, drained
- 2 cans chipotle peppers, finely chopped
- 1 tsp. chili powder
- ½ tsp. dried oregano
- ¼ tsp. ground cumin
- Pinch of sea salt, add more if needed
- Pinch of black pepper, to taste
- ½ avocado, sliced

Directions:
1. Heat the olive oil in a saucepan. Saute garlic, onion, mushrooms, zucchini, and red bell pepper for 5 minutes or until cooked through.

2. Add in tomatoes, pinto beans, chipotle peppers, chili powder, oregano, and cumin. Season with salt and pepper.

3. Reduce the heat to low and allow to simmer for 20 minutes or until beans are cooked through.

4. To serve, ladle soup into bowls. Top with avocado slices.

Dinner - Chicken and Mushroom Curry

Ingredients:

Garnishes, all optional

- 1 lime, sliced into wedges
- ⅛ cup fresh cilantro, minced

For the Garam masala

- 1 tsp. Spanish paprika powder
- 2 Tbsp. curry powder
- ¼ tsp. cinnamon powder
- ¼ tsp. oregano powder
- 1½ tsp. turmeric powder
- ½ tsp. cumin powder
- ½ tsp. coriander powder
- ¼ tsp. red pepper flakes
- ¼ tsp. black pepper

For the Aromatics

- 1 Tbsp. olive oil
- 1 onion, minced
- 3 garlic cloves, minced
- 1 ginger, minced
- 1 tomato, minced
- 1 lemongrass bulb, crushed

- 1 dried kefir lime leaf

For the Stew
- 2 lbs. chicken thighs, bone-in
- 1 sweet potato, cubed
- 1 can whole button mushrooms
- 1 red bell pepper, cubed
- 1 cup vegetable stock, low sodium
- 2 cans coconut cream, divided
- 1 birds' eye chili, halved lengthwise
- Pinch of sea salt, add more if needed
- Pinch of and black pepper, to taste
- water

Directions:
1. For the garam masala, put together Spanish paprika powder, curry powder, cinnamon powder, oregano powder, turmeric powder, cumin powder, coriander powder, red pepper flakes, and black pepper in a small bottle with tight-fitting lid.
2. Secure the lid and then shake well. Set aside.
3. Meanwhile, heat the olive oil in a pan. Once the oil is hot, saute onion, garlic, and ginger for 3 minutes or until limp and translucent.

Add in tomato, lemongrass, and kefir. Saute for 2 minutes.

4. Pour contents of the skillet onto the slow cooker.

5. For the stew, put chicken thighs, sweet potato, button mushrooms, and red bell pepper into the slow cooker.

6. Pour vegetable stock and coconut cream. Season with salt and pepper. Add in Stir in 1 tablespoon of garam masala.

7. Pour just enough water to cover all ingredients. Secure the lid and lock in place. Cook for 6 hours, undisturbed.

8. Pour the last can of coconut cream and bird's eye chili. Adjust taste if needed. Cook for another 30 minutes.

9. To serve, ladle into bowls. Garnish with cilantro. Squeeze in lime juice before eating.

Snacks/Desserts/Beverages

Carnation Flower Tisane

Ingredients:

- 1 cup water, at near boiling point
- 1 sprig mint
- 1 tsp. heaping carnation flower
- ¼ tsp. green stevia

Directions:

1. Pour water, mint, and carnation flower in a mug.
2. Allow to steep for 10 minutes. Strain the tea.
3. Serve with stevia.

Day 7

Breakfast - Plantains with Coconut Cream

Ingredients:

- 2 large plantains, overripe, unpeeled, boiled for 20 minutes, diced
- ½ cup canned coconut cream
- 1 Tbsp. desiccated coconut, toasted

Directions:

1. Pour coconut cream into a saucepan. Stir continuously until the cream thickens and turn into cream brown. Remove from heat.
2. Stirring often, cook until cream browns a little and thickens. Remove from heat.
3. Tip in plantains. Transfer to a bowl. Sprinkle toasted desiccated coconut on top. Serve.

Lunch - Salmon in Sauce

Ingredients:

- 2 tsp. extra-virgin olive oil
- ½ tsp. ground cumin
- Pinch of salt, add more if needed
- ½ tsp. black pepper
- ½ tsp. sugar
- 4 salmon fillets
- ½ cup Greek yogurt, non-fat
- 1 scallion, finely chopped
- 1 pickling cucumber, diced
- 3 tbsp. fresh parsley, minced
- 8 oz of whole wheat orzo, prepare according to package directions
- 1 teaspoon of fresh lemon juice

Directions:

1. Preheat the broiler.
2. Put together olive oil, cumin, salt, black pepper, and sugar in a mixing bowl. Stir well.
3. Line a baking sheet with tin foil. Layer the salmon fillets in the baking sheet. Grease the top of each fillet with the olive oil mixture. Place inside the fridge for 30 minutes.

4. Meanwhile, in another small bowl, combine yogurt, scallion, cucumber, parsley, lemon juice, and salt. Stir well.
5. Broil the salmon for 10 minutes or until opaque. Serve on top of the orzo with the yogurt sauce.

Dinner - Baked Snapper

Ingredients:
- 1 snapper fillet
- Pinch of sea salt, add more if needed
- Dash of smoky paprika
- 1 stalk fresh cilantro, minced

For the toppings
- ¼ tsp. capers in brine
- ½ cup frozen peas, thawed
- ½ cup fennel bulb, shaved thinly
- ¼ tsp. balsamic vinegar
- 1 tsp. lemon, freshly squeezed
- ⅛ tsp. dried pepper flakes
- Pinch of sea salt, add more if needed

Directions:
1. Preheat the oven to 450°F. Line a baking sheet with parchment paper.
2. Put together capers in brine, peas, fennel bulb, balsamic vinegar, lemon dried pepper flakes, and salt in a bowl. Set aside.

3. Season fish fillet with salt, paprika, and cilantro. Layer on a baking sheet. Bake for 10 minutes. Remove from the oven.

4. Pour topping mixture over the fish fillet. Bake for another 10 minutes.

5. Slide fish fillet in a serving platter. Serve.

Boiled Plantains with Berries, Raisins, and Walnuts

- 8 pieces overripe plantains
- water for boiling

For the Coconut cream sauce
- 1 can coconut cream
- 2 Tbsp. coconut sugar
- ¼ cup water
- Pinch of sea salt, add more if needed
- 1 drop vanilla extract

For the Seasonings
- ¼ cup raisins
- ½ cup berries of choice
- ¼ cup walnuts, roasted, chopped

Directions:
1. Layer plantains in a pot and cover with water.
2. Bring to a boil. Reduce the heat. Secure the lid and cook for 20 minutes or until plantains are cooked through.
3. Drain. Allow to cool before peeling and dicing.

4. For the coconut cream sauce, except for vanilla extract, pour coconut cream, coconut sugar, water, and salt into the saucepan.
5. Bring to a soft boil. Add in vanilla extract. Set aside.
6. To serve, put desired amount of plantains into a bowl. Sprinkle raisins, berries, and walnuts. Pour coconut cream sauce. Serve.

Day 8

Breakfast - Asparagus and Tuna Omelet

Ingredients:

- 3 eggs, whisked
- 1 can canned tuna flakes in oil, drained
- 3 asparagus, sliced thinly
- 1 pinch chives, minced
- Pinch of garlic salt, add more if needed
- Pinch of black pepper, to taste
- 1 Tbsp. olive oil

Directions:

1. Put together eggs, tuna flakes, asparagus, chives, garlic salt, and pepper into a bowl. Set aside.
2. Meanwhile, pour olive oil into the skillet. Once hot, pour the omelet mixture. Swirl the skillet to evenly distribute the ingredients.
3. Cook the eggs until the middle is no longer wobbly and the edges are set.
4. Remove from the skillet. Slice and serve.

Lunch - Greens and Blue Cheese Salad

Ingredients:
- 1 tsp. sour cream
- 1 tsp. blue cheese
- 1 tsp. apple cider vinegar
- Pinch of white pepper, to taste
- ¼ cup alfalfa sprouts
- 1 broccoli, sliced into bite-sized florets, steamed
- 1 cup iceberg lettuce, torn
- ½ tsp. cashew nuts, roasted

Directions:
1. Combine sour cream, blue cheese, apple cider and white pepper in a bowl. Whisk until the mixture is smooth and creamy. Set aside.
2. Meanwhile, in a salad bowl, put together alfalfa sprouts, broccoli lettuce, and cashew nuts. Toss well to combine.
3. Drizzle in blue cheese mixture into the leafy greens. Serve.

Dinner - Stir-Fried Pork Tenderloin

Ingredients:

- ½ pound pork tenderloin tips
- 1 tsp. sesame oil, divided
- Pinch of sea salt, add more if needed
- Pinch of white pepper
- 1 tsp. almond flour
- 1 white onion, julienned
- 1 red bell pepper, julienned
- 1 chili pepper, deseeded, julienned

Directions:

1. Marinade pork tenderloin with salt, white pepper, and almond flour. Set aside for 30-45 minutes.
2. Meanwhile, pour half of the sesame oil into a non-stick skillet. Stir-fry pork tenderloin for 4 minutes or until golden brown. Set aside.
3. In the same pan, pour the remaining sesame oil. Saute onion, red bell pepper, and chili pepper for 3 minutes or until fragrant and wilted.

4. Put the tenderloin back into pan. Continue cooking for 4 more minutes. Serve.

Snacks/Desserts/Beverages

Frozen Yogurt with Diced Fruits

Ingredients:
- 1 tub Greek yogurt
- 1 mango, diced
- 1 peach, diced
- 1 banana, diced
- 1 cup fresh berries of choice

Directions:
1. Fold diced mangoes, peach, banana, and fresh berries in a bowl. Put Greek yogurt. Gently toss to combine.
2. Scoop portions into freezer-safe containers. Freeze for 8 hours or overnight before serving.

Day 9

Breakfast - Asparagus Dipped in Soft Boiled Eggs

Ingredients:

- 2 eggs
- ¼ lb fresh asparagus
- water, for boiling
- Pinch of sea salt, add more if needed

Directions:

1. Pour water over the saucepan, half-filling it. Bring to a boil.
2. Lower the eggs onto the boiling water. Cook for 3 minutes.
3. Remove the eggs from the water. Set eggs side up into the egg cups.
4. Meanwhile, lower asparagus in the same boiling water. Cook until the asparagus turns a shade brighter. Remove from the heat
5. Strain out the cooked asparagus. Transfer to a serving plate lined with paper towels.
6. To serve, slice off the top of the eggs. Sprinkle little amount of salt. Dunk asparagus spears into the eggs. Enjoy!

Lunch - Chicken Soup

Ingredients:
- 1 Tbsp. olive oil
- 1 onion, minced
- ¼ lb. chicken thigh fillets, minced
- ½ tsp. chili powder
- 1 tsp. cumin powder
- ½ tsp. black pepper
- 1 fresh jalapeño pepper, minced
- Pinch of sea salt, add more if needed
- 1 can diced tomatoes
- 3 cups chicken broth, unsalted
- ½ just ripe avocado, sliced into thick half-moons, for garnish
- Pinch fresh cilantro, minced, for garnish

Directions:
1. Pour olive oil into a large saucepan. Saute onion, chicken, chili powder, cumin, black pepper, jalapeño, and salt for 10 minutes until the chicken has lost its pinkness. Stir continuously.
2. Add in tomatoes and pour chicken broth. Stir well.

3. Bring soup to a boil. Once boiling, reduce the heat and allow to simmer for 15 minutes.

4. Remove from heat. Let cool. Ladle desired amount of soup into bowls. Place avocado slices on the side. Garnish with cilantro on top. Serve.

Dinner - Spiced Chicken with Collard Greens

Ingredients:

- 2 chicken thigh fillets, pounded thin
- ½ cup sour cream
- 1 Tbsp. almond flour, finely milled, add more as needed
- Dash of cinnamon powder
- Dash of cayenne pepper powder
- Dash of black pepper
- Pinch of sea salt, add more if needed
- Pinch of white pepper, to taste
- Olive oil
- 1 lb. collard greens, chopped
- 3 garlic cloves, crushed
- water, for boiling

Directions:

1. Put together sour cream, cinnamon, cayenne, salt, and black pepper in a bowl. Place chicken thigh fillets and marinate for 1 hour. Set aside.
2. Strain out chicken fillets. Drain. Dredge fillets in almond flour. Make sure they are coated well.

3. Pour olive oil into a non-stick skillet. Fry chicken fillets for 8 minutes or until golden brown.
4. Damp on paper towels. Allow to cool for 5 minutes.
5. Meanwhile, in a saucepan, half-fill with water. Stir in garlic cloves. Bring to a boil. Tip in collard greens. Cook for 7 minutes or until the leaves turn dark and wilted. Drain.
6. Season with salt and pepper. Serve with cooked chicken.

Desserts/Snacks/Beverages

Kale Juice

Ingredients:

- 2 kale leaves
- 1 green apple, cored
- 1 beet, peeled
- 2 Swiss chard
- 1 lemon, halved
- 1 sprig mint

Directions:

1. Combine kale leaves, green apple, beet, Swiss chard, lemon, and sprig mint into a juicer. Process until all ingredients are well combined.
2. Transfer to a tall glass. Serve.

Day 10

Breakfast - Potted Eggs with Spinach

Ingredients

- ¼ tsp. olive oil, divided
- 1 garlic clove, minced
- ½ shallot, chopped
- 1 cup baby spinach leaves
- ½ cup, canned button mushrooms, drained
- ¼ cup single cream
- ¼ tsp. cheddar cheese, grated
- 1 egg
- Pinch of sea salt, add more if needed
- Pinch of pepper, to taste
- Dash of nutmeg powder

Directions:

1. Preheat the oven to 350°F. Lightly grease a ramekin with olive oil.
2. Pour remaining olive oil in a pan. Sauté garlic and shallot for 3 minutes or until aromatic and translucent.

3. Add in spinach and mushrooms. Cook for 2 minutes or until the spinach are wilted and the mushrooms are lightly cooked.

4. Pour into ramekin. Put a dollop of cream. Crack the egg. Season with salt, pepper cheese, and nutmeg powder.

5. Place ramekin in the middle rack of the oven. Bake for 10 minutes.

6. Remove from the oven. Serve.

Lunch - Pork Tenderloin with Tart Cherry Sauce

Ingredients:

- 4 tsp. olive oil, divided
- ¾ lbs. pork tenderloin, sliced into thick medallions
- 1 onion, minced
- ¼ cup dried tart cherries
- ¾ cup chicken broth, low-sodium
- 2 Tbsp. vinegar
- Pinch of sea salt, add more if needed
- Pinch of white pepper, to taste

Directions:

1. Season pork tenderloin with salt and white pepper. Set aside for 30 – 45 minutes.
2. Pour olive oil into a nonstick skillet. Once the oil is hot, cook pork medallions for 5 minutes until seared on both sides. Set aside cooked meat.
3. In the same skillet, pour the remaining olive oil. Saute onions for 2 minutes or until translucent.

4. Add in tart cherries, chicken broth, vinegar, salt, and pepper. Cook until the liquid is reduced by half.

5. Serve by placing pork medallions on top. Pour cherry sauce on top.

Dinner - Cauliflower Soup

Ingredients:

- 2 cups cauliflowers, sliced into bite-sized florets
- 1 sweet potato, diced
- 1 cup yellow summer squash, diced
- 2 cups fresh spinach, chopped
- 2 cups almond milk
- 2 cups vegetable stock
- ¼ cup almond cheese
- Pinch of sea salt, add more if needed
- Pinch of black pepper, to taste
- 1 Tbsp. fresh parsley, minced

Directions:

1. Pour vegetable stock in a large saucepan. Add in cauliflower florets, sweet potato, and squash. Secure the lid. Bring mixture to a rolling boil.
2. Once boiling, reduce the heat and allow to simmer for 15 minutes or until the vegetables are cooked through.

3. Cook spinach leaves for 1 minute. Pour almond milk, vegetable stock, almond cheese, salt, and pepper. Stir well.
4. To serve, ladle soup into bowls. Garnish with parsley. Serve.

Desserts/Snacks/Beverages

Ginger Tea

Ingredients:

- 1 fresh ginger, crushed
- 1 cup water, near boiling point
- ¼ tsp. green stevia

Directions:

1. Put together ginger, water, and green stevia in a mug. Let the tea brew for 10 minutes.
2. Strain and then serve.

Day 11

Breakfast – Soft-Boiled Eggs on Layer of Greens

Ingredients:

For the dressing
- 1 tsp. Dijon mustard
- 4 tsp. apple cider vinegar
- 2 tsp. olive oil
- Pinch of sea salt, add more if needed
- Pinch of white pepper, to taste

For the salad
- 2 cups arugula leaves, torn
- ½ cup iceberg lettuce, torn
- 1 ripe tomato, minced
- ½ cup baby spinach leaves, torn
- 2 soft-boiled eggs, peeled

Directions:
1. Put together Dijon mustard, apple cider vinegar, olive oil, salt, and pepper into a bottle with tight-fitting lid. Shake well. Set aside.

2. Place arugula leaves, iceberg lettuce, tomato, and baby spinach in a salad bowl. Drizzle in just the right amount of dressing. Toss well to combine.

3. Spoon desired amount of greens on plates. Create a well in the center. Put a soft-boiled egg. Drizzle in remaining dressing. Break the eggs so that the yolks run into salad. Serve.

Lunch - Halibut with Peas and Beans

Ingredients:

- olive oil, for frying
- 2 halibut fillets, trimmed well
- Pinch of sea salt, add more if needed
- Pinch of white pepper, to taste
- ½ cup frozen peas, thawed
- 1 cup, French beans, halved
- ½ lime, sliced into wedges

Directions:

1. Season fillet with salt and pepper. Pour olive oil into a non-stick pan. Once the oil is hot, slide halibut fillets and cook for 5 minutes or until well seared on both sides.
2. Remove from the pan. Set aside on a plate and cover with aluminum foil.
3. In the same pan, pour the remaining olive oil. Cook peas and French beans for 3 minutes or until the veggies turn a shade brighter.
4. To serve, put fish at the center and place greens on the side. Squeeze in lime juice.

Dinner – Three-Cheese Salad

Ingredients:
- 1 head iceberg lettuce, chopped
- 1 unripe tomato, sliced
- 1 stalk parsley, torn
- 1 jalapeño pepper, julienned
- 2 balls mozzarella, quartered
- 1 tsp. cottage cheese
- 1 tsp. edam cheese, grated
- 1 tsp. apple cider vinegar

Directions:
1. Put together iceberg lettuce, tomato, parsley, jalapeño pepper, mozzarella, cottage cheese, and edam cheese in a salad bowl.
2. Season with apple cider vinegar. Toss well. Serve.

Desserts/Snacks/Beverages

Fried Plantains with Sesame Seeds and Walnuts

Ingredients:

- 2 ripe plantains, sliced diagonally into thick medallions
- 1 Tbsp. coconut oil
- ½ cup shelled walnuts, chopped, toasted
- ½ tsp. sesame seeds, toasted

Directions:

1. Pour coconut oil into a non-stick skillet. Cook plantain slices until golden brown on both sides.
2. Transfer to a serving plate. Damp with paper towels. Repeat cooking step until all of plantains are cooked.
3. Garnish with sesame seeds and walnuts on top. Serve.

Day 12

Breakfast - Egg Salad on Cucumber Disks

For the Homemade Mayonnaise

- 2 egg yolks
- 1 cup extra virgin olive oil
- 4 tsp. lemon juice, freshly-squeezed
- 1 tsp. Dijon mustard
- Pinch of sea salt, add more if needed

For the egg salad
- 1 Tbsp. homemade mayonnaise
- Pinch of sea salt, add more if needed
- Pinch of white pepper, to taste
- Dash of Spanish paprika
- 2 eggs, hardboiled, separate whites from yolks

For the cucumber disks
- 4 cucumber disks, sliced diagonally
- Pinch of salt, add more if needed
- Pinch of black pepper, to taste
- 1 Tbsp. apple cider vinegar

Directions:

1. For the mayonnaise, combine lemon juice and salt in a bowl. Whisk until the salt dissolves.

2. Meanwhile, pour mustard and egg yolks in a blender. Pulse until all ingredients are well combined.

3. While the blender is running, pour oil in a slow, thin stream. Once the oil no longer separates from the other liquids, increase the amount of oil. Wait until the mayo thickens.

4. Place inside the fridge in an airtight container until ready to use.

5. For the egg salad: combine homemade mayonnaise salt pepper and paprika in a bowl. Place inside the fridge until ready to use.

6. For the cucumber disks, put together cucumber disks, salt, pepper, and apple cider vinegar in a bowl. Drain.

7. To serve, put cucumber disks on a platter. Scoop an equal amount of egg salad into the hollowed out egg whites. Place filling-side down on cucumber disks.

Lunch - Parmesan Crusted Tilapia

Ingredients:
- 2 tilapia fillets
- Pinch of sea salt, add more if needed
- Pinch of black pepper, to taste
- 1 Tbsp. steel-cut oats
- Pinch of oregano powder
- Pinch of garlic powder
- 1 Tbsp. parmesan cheese, grated
- olive oil, for shallow frying

Directions:
1. Season tilapia fillets with a salt and pepper. Set aside.
2. Place oats, oregano powder, garlic powder, and parmesan cheese in a blender. Process mixture until finely milled. Transfer to a bowl.
3. Roll tilapia fillets into the oatmeal mix. Make sure all sides are evenly coated.
4. Meanwhile, in a nonstick skillet, heat the olive oil. Once hot, fry the tilapia fillets for 5 minutes or until golden brown on both sides. Remove from the pan immediately. Serve.

Dinner - Stir-Fry Turkey Ham and Cauliflower

Ingredients:
- 1 Tbsp. olive oil
- 2 slices turkey ham, diced
- 1 head cauliflower, sliced into bite-sized florets
- Dash of cumin powder
- 2 Tbsp. water
- Pinch of sea salt, add more if needed
- Pinch of black pepper, to taste

Directions:
1. Heat the olive oil in a nonstick skillet. Stir-fry turkey ham for 3 minutes or until lightly seared.
2. Add in cauliflower florets, cumin powder, water, salt, and pepper. Secure the lid. Cook for 6 minutes.
3. Turn off the heat. Transfer contents of the pan to a serving plate. Serve.

Snacks/Desserts/Beverages

Spiced Sweet Potato Matchsticks

Ingredients:

For the Spice mix
- ½ tsp. all spice powder
- Dash of ginger powder
- 1 tsp. cinnamon powder
- Dash of nutmeg powder
- Pinch of sea salt, add more if needed
- olive oil for drizzling
- 2 sweet potatoes, sliced into thick matchsticks

Directions:
1. Preheat the oven to 250°F. Line a baking sheet with aluminum foil.
2. Put together all spice powder, ginger powder, cinnamon powder, nutmeg powder, and salt in a small bowl.
3. Layer sweet potatoes flat on the baking sheet. Drizzle in olive oil. Place inside the oven and bake for 2 hours. Flip sweet potatoes midway through baking.

4. Transfer baked sweet potatoes into the spice mixture. Toss well to combine. Serve.

Day 13

Breakfast - Eggs Florentine

Ingredients:

- 1 cup spinach, chopped
- 1/2 cup low fat cheese
- 5 eggs
- Pinch of sea salt, add more if needed
- Pinch of pepper, to taste

Directions:

1. Season spinach with salt and pepper. Layer them on the non-stick skillet. Add water.
2. Once partly cooked, crack in eggs on top. Season with salt and pepper.
3. Once set, sprinkle cheese. Allow the cheese to melt before removing from the pan.
4. Slide in a serving platter. Serve.

Lunch - Beef and Veggie Stew

For the Stew

- 2 lbs. bone in beef shin, sliced in manageable portions
- 1 fresh ginger, crushed
- 2 onions, quartered
- 2 cups beef stock
- water
- 1 dried bay leaf
- Pinch of sea salt, add more if needed
- 1 tsp. whole black peppercorns
- 1 green cabbage, quartered
- 1 handful bok choi, sliced into long slivers

Directions:

1. Combine beef shin, ginger, onions, beef stock, water, bay leaf, salt, and pepper in a slow cooker. Make sure all ingredients are submerged in liquid.
2. Secure the lid and lock in place. Cook for 6 hours, undisturbed. Discard bay leaf and ginger.

3. Add in bok choi and cabbage. Secure the lid and cook for another 30 minutes. Adjust seasoning if needed.
4. Ladle into bowls. Serve.

Dinner - **Seafood Soup**

Ingredients:
- Pinch of parsley, minced

For the aromatics
- 2 Tbsp. olive oil
- 1 onion, minced
- 2 garlic cloves, minced
- 1 fennel bulb, julienned
- 2 celery stalks, minced
- ½ tsp. red pepper flakes
- 1 tsp. powdered oregano
- Pinch of sea salt, add more if needed
- Pinch of black pepper, to taste
- 2 bay leaves, whole

For the Liquids
- 1 can whole clams in clam juice, liquid reserved
- 1 can tomatoes, crushed
- ½ Tbsp. tomato paste
- 3 cups fish stock

For the Seafood

- ½ pound frozen halibut fillets, thawed, cubed
- 1 pound green-lipped mussels, scrubbed clean
- ½ pound frozen prawns, thawed
- 1 pound neck clams, soaked in salted water for 1 hour
- ½ pound frozen squid rings, thawed

Directions:

1. Pour olive oil into a large saucepan. Once the oil is hot, sauté onion and garlic for 3 minutes or until limp and fragrant. Do not burn the garlic.
2. Add in fennel bulb, celery stalks, red pepper flakes, oregano, salt, pepper, and bay leaf into the mixture. Stir continuously.
3. Pour whole clams with juice, crushed tomatoes tomato paste, and fish stock. Bring mixture to a rolling boil. Cook for 5 minutes or until the liquid is reduced by half.
4. Add in halibut fillets, mussels, prawns, neck clams, and squid rings. Cover and allow to simmer for another 5 minutes.

5. Discard bay leaf and shells that did not open. Season with salt and pepper.
6. Garnish with parsley. Serve.

Snacks/Desserts/Beverages

Peanut Butter Cup

Ingredients:

- 1 tablespoon cocoa powder, unsweetened
- 1 tablespoon chocolate protein powder, plant-based
- ½ cup almond milk, unsweetened
- ½ tablespoon peanut butter, natural, unsalted
- Water

Directions:

1. Put together cocoa powder, chocolate protein powder, almond milk, and peanut butter in food processor. Process until all ingredients are well-combined.
2. Add water and continue pulsing until a desired consistency is achieved.
3. Pour in a tall glass. Serve.

Day 14

Breakfast - Egg Cups

Ingredients:
- 6 streaky bacon strips
- 3 eggs
- 2 green beans, sliced diagonally
- Pinch of sea salt, add more if needed
- Pinch of black pepper, to taste
- Dried chili flakes, optional

Directions:
1. Preheat the oven to 400°F. Put 3 laminated paper liners into 3 muffin tins. Put green beans into the paper liners.
2. Layer 2 bacon strips on the side of the paper liner. Make sure to overhang bacon so that they won't fold during the baking process.
3. Crack an egg into the muffin tin. Season with salt and pepper. Bake for 12 minutes or until the bacon is crisp and the eggs are set.
4. Remove muffin tin from the oven. Serve egg cups in paper liners.

Lunch – Pumpkin and Tomato Soup

Ingredients:

- 1 tablespoon olive oil
- 1 onion, chopped
- 4 garlic cloves, pressed
- 2 celery stalks, chopped
- 1 cup pumpkin, chopped
- 1 tomato, chopped
- 1 red bell pepper, chopped
- 1 tablespoon Spanish paprika
- ½ teaspoon cinnamon powder
- 3 tablespoons turmeric
- Pinch of sea salt, add more if needed
- Pinch of pepper, to taste
- 1 bay leaf
- ½ teaspoon hot sauce

Directions:

1. In a large saucepan, heat the olive oil. Once the oil is hot, saute onion, garlic, and celery for 5 minutes or until limp and aromatic.

2. Add in pumpkin, tomato, red bell pepper, Spanish paprika, cinnamon powder,

turmeric, salt, pepper, bay leaf, and hot sauce. Cook for 3 minutes whilst stirring continuously. Serve.

Dinner – Basil-Flavored Chicken

Ingredients:

- 1 lb. chicken meat, cubed
- Pinch of sea salt, add more if needed
- Pinch of pepper, to taste
- 3 tablespoons olive oil
- 2 garlic cloves, minced
- 1 red bell pepper, chopped
- 2 cups zucchini, sliced
- 1 cup mushrooms, sliced
- ½ cup basil, chopped, divided

Directions:

1. Season the chicken meat with salt, pepper, and basil.
2. Meanwhile, heat the olive oil in a pan. Once the oil is hot, saute garlic for 2 minutes.
3. Add in seasoned chicken meat, red bell pepper, zucchini, mushrooms, and basil.
4. Cook for 5 minutes or until the chicken is cooked through and the veggies tender. Serve.

Snacks/Desserts/Beverages

Jalapeno Cheddar Poppers

Ingredients:

- 1 spring roll wrapper cut in half
- 1 egg
- 2 jalapeno peppers, halved lengthwise
- Cheddar cheese, low fat, sliced into strips

Directions:

1. Brush spring roll wrapper with egg.
2. Meanwhile, put together jalapeño peppers and cheese strips in a bowl.
3. Place the mixture on the spring roll wrapper. Fold and roll the edges.
4. Heat the oil in a pan. Cook poppers for 3 minutes or until the wrapper is brown and the cheese has melted. Serve.

Chapter 3
Phases 2 and 3 Recipes

Breakfast Recipes

Strawberry and Peanut Butter Oats Bowl

Ingredients:
- 1 cup water
- 1 tablespoon peanut butter, natural
- ½ cup quick-cooking oats
- ½ cup strawberries

Directions:
1. Pour water into a large saucepan. Fill with water and bring to a boil.
2. Once the water is boiling, stir in quick-cooking oats and stir. Cook for 3 minutes.
3. Add in peanut butter and strawberries into the mixture. Stir well until all ingredients are well-combined. Serve.

Almond Pancakes with Coconut Flakes

Ingredients:

For the garnish
- ¼ cup coconut flakes, sweetened
- 2 Tbsp. almond flakes, blanched
- Dash of cinnamon powder
- Pinch of sea salt, add more if needed
- Pure maple syrup, use sparingly

For the Almond Pancakes
- 2 eggs, yolks and whites separated
- 1 cup almond flour, finely milled
- 1 banana, overripe preferred, mashed
- ½ cup applesauce, unsweetened
- ¼ cup water
- ¼ tsp. coconut oil

Directions:
1. For the garnish, preheat the oven to 350°F. Line a baking sheet with parchment paper. Set aside.
2. Meanwhile, put together coconut and almond flakes in a bowl. Spread on the baking sheet. Bake for 10 minutes.

3. Remove from the oven. Allow the mixture to cool before putting cinnamon powder and salt. Set aside.

4. For the pancakes, beat egg whites until soft peaks form.

5. Combine egg yolks, almond flour, banana, applesauce, and water in another bowl. Mix well until all ingredients are well combined. Fold in egg whites.

6. Pour olive oil into a nonstick skillet. Once the oil is hot, pour just the right amount of batter. Cook until bubbles form in the center and the edges are set. Serve.

Grapefruit and Kiwi Cold Brew

Ingredients:

- 4 cups water
- 2 kiwi fruits, quartered
- 1 grapefruit, torn into large chunks
- 1 lemon, quartered

Directions:

1. Pour water in a pitcher. Add in kiwi fruits, grapefruit, and lemon. Secure the lid.
2. Place inside the fridge for 4 – 6 hours. Stir mixture every hour.
3. Strain brew before serving. Serve chilled.

Purple Coconut Flapjacks

Ingredients:
- 2 eggs, yolks and whites separated
- 1 cup coconut flour, finely milled
- 1 banana, preferably overripe, mashed
- ½ cup blueberries
- ¼ cup water
- ¼ tsp. coconut oil

Directions:
1. Whisk egg whites until soft peaks form. Set aside.
2. Meanwhile, put together egg yolks, coconut flour, banana, half of blueberries, and water in a bowl. Mix until all ingredients are well incorporated. Fold in egg whites.
3. Heat the coconut oil in a nonstick skillet. Once the oil is hot, pour just the right amount of batter. Cook until bubbles form in the center and the edges are set. Serve.

Blueberries and Mango Oats

Ingredients:
- ¼ cup steel-cut oats, cooked
- 1 mango cheek, diced into bite-sized piece
- ¼ cup frozen blueberries

Directions:
1. Combine blueberries and cooked oats in a bowl. Mash berries. Add in diced mangoes. Serve warm.

Blackberry and Lemon Thyme Tea

Ingredients:

- 4 cups water
- 1 cup frozen blackberries
- 1 lemon, sliced into wedges
- 1 fresh thyme sprig

Directions:

1. Pour water in a saucepan. Add in blackberries. Secure the loid and bring mixture to a boil.
2. Reduce the heat and allow to simmer for 10 minutes. Turn off the heat.
3. Add in lemon wedges and thyme sprigs. Allow to steep for 5 minutes.
4. To serve, put lemon disks into cups. Pour herbal infusion. Top with bits of blackberries.

Plantain Hash with Soft Boiled Egg and Bacon

Ingredients:

- ½ tsp. olive oil
- 8 streaky bacon
- 2 eggs, soft-boiled
- 1 plantain, ripe, sliced into thick disks
- ½ pound fresh kale, chopped
- Pinch of sea salt, add more if needed
- Pinch of black pepper, to taste

Directions:

1. Pour olive oil into a non-stick skillet. Once the oil is hot, fry bacon until crispy. Drain on paper towels.
2. Fry plantains until golden brown. Reduce the heat and cook kale leaves. Season with salt and pepper. Stir well.
3. To serve, put plantain hash into plates. Serve with soft boiled eggs and bacon on the side.

Chicken and Waffles

Ingredients:

For the chicken
- 2 cups olive oil, for deep frying
- ½ cup almond flour, finely milled
- 1 pound chicken thighs, bone-in
- Pinch of sea salt, add more if needed
- Pinch of white pepper, to taste

For the waffles
- olive oil, for greasing
- ½ cup almond flour, finely milled
- ½ tsp. baking powder
- 2 eggs, whisked
- ½ tsp. vanilla extract

Directions:
1. Season chicken thighs with salt and pepper. Set aside in a colander and place inside the fridge for 30 minutes.
2. After 30 minutes, coat chicken thighs with almond flour.

3. Meanwhile, heat the olive oil in a skillet. Once the oil is hot, cook coated and marinated chicken thighs for 5 minutes or until golden brown. Drain on paper towels.

4. For the waffles, preheat the waffle iron. Lightly grease waffle iron with olive oil.

5. Put together almond flour, baking powder, eggs, and vanilla extract in a bowl. Mix until just mixed.

6. Spoon an equal amount of batter into the waffle iron. Cook until firm. Repeat the same cooking procedure until all batter are cooked and used up.

7. To serve, put waffles and chicken on plates.

Chia Seed Bread

Ingredients:

Dry ingredients
- ½ cup coconut flour, finely milled
- 1 tsp. baking powder
- 2 Tbsp. chia seeds, ground
- Pinch of sea salt, add more if needed

Wet ingredients
- 6 eggs, whites and yolks separated, whites whisk until soft peaks form
- ½ cup coconut milk
- 4 Tbsp. coconut butter
- 1 tsp. apple cider vinegar

Directions:
1. Preheat the oven to 350°F. Line a bread loaf pan with parchment paper. Grease paper with coconut butter. Set aside.
2. Sift coconut flour, baking powder, chai seeds, and sea salt thrice. Transfer to mixing bowl. Create a well in the center.

3. Pour coconut milk, coconut butter, and apple cider vinegar into the well. Mix until all ingredients are well-combined. Fold in whisked egg whites.

4. Pour batter into the loaf pan. Put aluminum foil but make sure that it is loose.

5. Bake the bread for 30 minutes. Remove the aluminum foil without removing the pan from the oven. Bake for another 10 minutes or until golden brown.

6. Brush the tops with melted coconut butter. Allow the cake to cool on a cake rack before slicing.

Poppy Seed Bread

Ingredients:

Wet ingredients
- 1 lemon, juiced and zested
- ¼ cup raw organic honey
- ¼ cup coconut oil, reserve some for greasing
- 1 egg

Dry ingredients
- ¼ tsp. baking soda
- ¼ cup coconut flour
- Pinch of sea salt, add more if needed
- 1 Tbsp. poppy seeds, reserve some for garnish

Directions:
1. Preheat the oven to 350°F. Line two mini loaf pans with parchment paper. Grease the paper. Set aside.
2. Pour lemon juice, honey, and coconut oil in a bowl. Mix well.
3. Pour in baking soda, coconut flour, and salt in another bowl. Mix well. Fold in poppy seeds.

4. Pour equal amounts of batter into the mini loaf pans. Sprinkle poppy seeds on top.
5. Bake for 20 minutes. Remove pans from the oven and allow to cool for 15 minutes before slicing and serving.

Lunch Recipes

Roasted Beef and Veggies

- 2½ lbs. beef bones, preferably with meat still attached
- 2 onions, halved
- ¼ butternut squash, cubed
- 1 red bell pepper, cubed
- 1 sweet potato, chopped
- olive oil, for drizzling
- 4 garlic heads, tops sliced off to expose cloves

Directions:

1. Preheat the oven to 350 degrees °F. Line a roasting tin and baking sheet with aluminum foil.
2. Layer beef bones in the roasting tin. Roast for 20 minutes or until browned all over. Flip and roast the other side for 10 minutes. Remove from the oven and set aside.
3. For the vegetables, put together onions, butternut squash, red bell pepper, and sweet potato in the baking sheet. Drizzle in olive oil. Toss well to combine.

4. Pour the mixture and make sure to spread evenly. Put the garlic heads in the corners. Season with salt. Roast for 20 minutes.

Microwave Asparagus

Ingredients:

- 2½ pounds, thick-stemmed white asparagus, sliced
- 2 Tbsp. olive oil
- Pinch of sea salt, add more if needed

Directions:

1. Layer asparagus in a microwave-safe dish. Drizzle in olive oil. Season with salt.
2. Cover dish with saran wrap. Place inside the microwave oven and cook for 10 seconds.
3. Remove saran wrap. Let cool before serving.

Chicken-Ginger Stew

Ingredients:

- ¼ cup chicken thigh fillet, diced
- 1 unripe papaya, peeled, diced
- 1 ginger, crushed
- ¼ cup egg noodles, cooked
- 1 cup chicken stock, low fat, low-sodium
- 1 cup water
- 1 tsp. fish sauce
- 1 bird's eye chili, minced
- Dash of garlic powder
- Dash of onion powder
- Pinch of white pepper

Directions:

1. Put together chicken thigh fillet, papaya, egg noodles, ginger, chicken stock, water fish sauce, bird's eye chili, garlic powder, onion powder, and white pepper in a large saucepan. Bring to a boil.
2. Once boiling, reduce the heat. Allow stew to simmer for 20 minutes or until the papaya is tender and the chicken fillet is cooked through. Serve hot.

Chicken and Mushroom Pot Pie

Ingredients:

- ¼ cup chicken, cooked, shredded
- 1 can mushroom pieces and stems
- ¼ cup frozen peas, thawed
- 2 Tbsp. milk, low fat
- ½ cup vegetable stock, low-sodium
- Pinch of sea salt, add more if needed
- Pinch of black pepper, to taste
- 1 package, puff pastry dough, rolled thin

Directions:

1. Preheat the oven to 400°F.
2. Put together shredded chicken, mushroom stems and pieces, peas, ilk, vegetable stock, salt, and pepper in a bowl.
3. Transfer to a ramekin and place puff pastry dough on top. Seal the edges and trim excess dough.
4. Bake for 20 minutes until the pastry turns brown. Remove from the oven. Serve.

Grilled Pepper and Sausages

Ingredients:

For the Mustard Spread
- 1 Tbsp. Dijon mustard
- 1 Tbsp. grainy mustard
- 3 Tbsp. homemade mayonnaise
- 1 Tbsp. parsley, minced
- 2 tsp. garlic powder
- 1 tsp. black pepper

For the Marinade and sausages
- 4 links Italian sausages
- 1 white onion, quartered
- 2 garlic cloves, crushed
- 1 red bell pepper, cubed
- 1 green bell pepper, cubed
- 2 Tbsp. fresh parsley, chopped
- 2 Tbsp. fresh oregano, chopped
- ¼ cup red wine vinegar
- Pinch of sea salt, add more if needed
- Pinch of black pepper, to taste
- ½ cup olive oil
- olive oil for brushing

Directions:

1. For the mustard, put together Dijon mustard, grainy mustard, mayonnaise, parsley, garlic powder, and black pepper in a bowl. Mix well until all ingredients are well-combined. Store in an airtight container until ready to use.

2. For the marinade and sausages: pour all ingredients into a freezer-safe freezer safe bag. Remove as much air from the bag and seal.

3. Massage ingredients gently to incorporate flavors but try not to separate onion wedges. Set aside for at least two hours before grilling.

4. Set grill pan over medium heat.

5. Fish out sausages, onion quarters, and bell pepper cubes. Drain lightly. Reserve marinade for basting.

6. Grill sausages, onions, and peppers for 5 minutes, loosely tented with a sheet of aluminum foil. Baste with marinade in $2\frac{1}{2}$ minute intervals. Flip, and grill other side for 5 more minutes.

7. Transfer cooked sausages and vegetables to a plate. Put a dollop of Spicy Mustard Spread on the side.

Steak Sandwich

Ingredients:

For the Steak
- ½ pound sirloin steak
- Pinch of sea salt, add more if needed
- Pinch of black pepper, to taste
- olive oil, for frying
- 1 Tbsp. grainy mustard

For the Salad
- 1 arugula
- 1 radish, sliced thinly
- ¼ cup alfalfa sprouts
- 1 tsp. fresh cranberries
- ¼ tsp. apple cider vinegar
- Pinch of sea salt, add more if needed
- Pinch of black pepper, to taste

Directions:
1. For the steak, season sirloin steak with salt and pepper. Wrap tightly in saran wrap. Place inside the fridge for 30 minutes. Drain the meat.

2. Lightly grease a pan with oil.

3. Wait for the oil to become smoky before frying the sirloin steak. Cook for 5 minutes. Flip the other side and cook for another 5 minutes. Turn off the heat.

4. Transfer to a plate. Allow the meat to rest for 10 minutes before slicing.

5. For the salad, combine arugula, alfalfa sprouts, cranberries, salt, and pepper in a bowl. Toss gently until combined.

6. To serve, spread the mustard on bread slices. Place a generous amount of salad on one bread slice and sliced steak. Top off with the other bread slice. Serve.

Tuna Salad

Ingredients:

For the salad

- 1 head watercress, torn
- ½ lb. baby spinach, torn
- 1 head iceberg lettuce, roughly torn

For the tuna salad:

- 1 green mango, minced
- 1 ripe mango, diced
- 1 red bird's eye chilli, minced
- 1 green banana chilli, minced
- 1 can tuna chunks in oil
- ½ cup cottage cheese
- 2 Tbsp. English mustard
- ¼ cup yogurt, low fat
- 1 tsp. fish sauce
- 1 lime, zested, juiced
- Pinch of sea salt, add more if needed
- Pinch of white pepper, to taste

Directions:

1. For the tuna salad, combine green mango, ripe mango, red bird's eye chili, green banana

chili, tuna chunks in oil, cottage cheese, mustard, yogurt, and fish sauce in a mixing bowl.

2. Drizzle in lime juice. Season with salt and pepper. Place inside the fridge to chill for 30 minutes.

3. To serve, place watercress, spinach, and lettuce in a bowl. Drizzle in a few drops of lime juice all over. Put an equal amount of salad on plates. Top with chilled tuna salad. Serve.

Sirloin Steak Beef with Vegetables

Ingredients:

For the steak
- ⅛ tsp. olive oil
- 1 beef sirloin steak, pounded, sliced into matchsticks
- ⅛ tsp. light soy sauce
- ⅛ tsp. flour
- Pinch of black pepper, to taste

For the salad
- ¼ Asian turnip, sliced into matchsticks
- 1 cucumber, sliced into matchsticks
- 1 stalk leek, white part only, sliced into matchsticks
- 1 radish, thinly shaved
- ⅛ tsp. apple cider vinegar
- Pinch of sea salt, add more if needed

Directions:
1. Pour olive oil into a non-stick skillet.
2. Combine beef sirloin, soy sauce, flour, and pepper in a bowl. Mix well.

3. Fry matchstick for 5 minutes or until golden brown. Remove from the pan.

4. For the salad, toss turnip, cucumber, leek, radish, apple cider vinegar, and salt in a salad bowl. Mix well.

5. To serve, place salad on a plate. Top with beef steak. Serve.

Dinner

Beef Bourguignon

Ingredients:

- 2 lbs. beef chuck roast, cubed
- Pinch of sea salt, add more if needed
- Pinch of white pepper, to taste
- 1 tsp. olive oil
- 1 onion, chopped
- 2 garlic cloves, minced
- 2 cups beef broth, low-sodium
- 1 cup dry red wine
- 1 dried bay leaf
- 1 tsp. thyme, chopped
- 1 lemon, sliced into wedges

Directions:

1. Preheat the oven to 300°F or 150°C for at least 10 minutes.
2. Meanwhile, pour olive oil into a large saucepan.
3. Season beef chuck with salt and white pepper. Fry in oil until golden brown on all sides.

Transfer partially cooked meat on a holding plate.

4. In the same saucepan, sauté onions and garlic. Sauté for 3 minutes or until limp and translucent.

5. Pour beef broth, dry red wine, bay leaf, and thyme. Add in beef cubes. Stir gently.

6. Place cookware into the oven. Slow cook for 4 hours.

7. After the 4-hour mark, remove from the oven. Serve with lemon wedge.

Mushroom Kabobs

Ingredients:
- 4 Tbsp. olive oil
- 4 garlic cloves, grated
- 2½ pounds button mushrooms
- ½ tsp. dried basil, crumbled
- ½ tsp. dried oregano, crumbled
- ½ cup balsamic vinegar
- 4 Tbsp. parsley, minced, for garnish
- 1 lime, sliced into wedges, for garnish

Directions:
1. Set grill pan over medium heat.
2. Combine garlic, button mushrooms, dried basil, oregano, and balsamic vinegar in a bowl. Transfer to a freezer-safe bag. Seal.
3. Massage ingredients and place inside the fridge for 20 minutes.
4. Drain mushrooms and reserve the marinade.
5. Thread mushrooms into a bamboo skewer. Repeat the same step for the remaining mushrooms.

6. Grill mushrooms for 10 minutes. Flip often until evenly cooked. Baste using the marinade.
7. Place mushrooms on a serving platter. Garnish with parsley. Serve.

Ensalada Valencia

Ingredients:
- 1 tsp. white wine vinegar
- 1 tsp. Dijon mustard
- 1 tsp. extra virgin olive oil
- Pinch of sea salt, add more if needed
- Pinch of black pepper, to taste
- Pinch of fresh thyme, minced
- 1 head Romaine lettuce, sliced into bite-sized pieces
- ½ tangerine, pulp only
- ½ onion, julienned
- 1 tsp. Kalamata olives in oil, julienned

Directions:
1. Combine white wine vinegar, Dijon mustard, extra virgin olive oil, salt, pepper, and fresh thyme. Whisk well until the dressing emulsifies.
2. Toss together Romaine lettuce, tangerine, onion, and olives in salad bowl.
3. Drizzle in dressing all over salad. Serve.

Pork Tenderloin with Grape Vinaigrette

Ingredients:

For the grape vinaigrette
- ¼ cup red grapes, quartered
- ¼ cup green grapes, quartered
- 1 tsp. apple cider vinegar
- black peppercorns, cracked
- 1 medallion pork tenderloin
- Pinch of sea salt, add more if needed
- 1 tsp. sesame oil

Directions:
1. For the vinaigrette, combine red and green grapes, apple cider vinegar, and peppercorns in a bowl. Chill.
2. Season pork with salt and sesame oil. Grill for 12 minutes.
3. Remove from the grill. Place aluminum foil and allow to rest for 5 minutes.
4. Transfer to a plate. Drizzle in vinaigrette. Serve.

Coconut Shrimp with Chayote

Ingredients:

- 2 Tbsp. coconut oil
- 2 garlic clove, grated
- 1 onion, minced
- 1 tsp. ginger, grated
- ½ cup shrimp stock
- 2 cans coconut cream
- 3 chayote, peeled, sliced into flat ribbons using a spiralizer
- 2½ lb. shrimp
- 2 bird's eye chili, halved lengthwise
- 1 tsp. Spanish paprika powder
- Pinch of sea salt, add more if needed
- Pinch of white pepper, to taste
- Pinch of cilantro, minced, for garnish

Directions:

1. Pour coconut oil into the Dutch oven.
2. Saute garlic, onions, and ginger for 3 minutes or until limp and aromatic.
3. Pour shrimp stock and coconut cream. Bring mixture to a rolling boil.

4. Reduce the heat and let it simmer for 20 minutes. Add in chayote and shrimp. Cook for 5 minutes or only until the shrimps turn coral.

5. Turn off heat. Stir in bird's eye chili, paprika powder, salt, and pepper. Garnish with cilantro. Serve.

Sweet and Sour Meatballs

Ingredients:

For the Meatballs
- coconut oil, for greasing
- 2½ pounds ground beef
- 1 Tbsp. coconut flour, finely milled
- 2 eggs, whisked
- ¼ cup cilantro, minced
- ½ cup chives, minced
- Pinch of sea salt, add more if needed
- Pinch of black pepper, to taste

For the Sauce
- 1 banana chili, julienned
- 1 red bell pepper, julienned
- ¼ cup tomato sauce
- 1 tsp. tomato paste
- ¼ cup coconut vinegar
- 2 Tbsp. coconut sugar
- ¼ cup water
- Pinch of sea salt, add more if needed
- Pinch of white pepper, to taste

Directions:

1. Preheat the oven to 400 degrees °F for the meatballs. Lightly grease saucepan with coconut oil.

2. Combine ground beef, coconut flour, eggs, cilantro, chives, salt, and pepper in a bowl. Roll into meatballs and place inside the saucepan.

3. Cook for 10 minutes, flipping the other side halfway through the cooking process. Turn off the heat.

4. Put together banana chili, red bell pepper tomato sauce tomato paste coconut vinegar, coconut sugar, water, salt, and pepper in another bowl. Pour sauce over meatballs.

5. Put the lid on and cook in the oven for 40 minutes.

6. Remove from the oven. Let residual heat cook the meal further.

7. To serve, ladle desired amount of meatballs into a bowl.

Snacks/Desserts/Beverages

Green Tea with Fresh Strawberries

Ingredients:

- 1 lb. fresh strawberries, halved
- 4 cups water
- ¼ cup basil
- 4 teabags green tea

Directions:

1. Place strawberries, water, basil, and green tea teabags into a large pitcher. Mix gently bruising fruits and herbs. Place inside the fridge to chill for 4 hours.
2. Discard herbs and teabags. Serve chilled.

Garlic and Sundried Tomato Bread

Ingredients:

- 2 sugar-free sourdough bread, toasted
- 1 garlic clove, peeled
- 2 tsp. sun dried tomatoes in olive oil, minced
- 1 tsp. olive oil
- 1 tsp. chives, minced

Directions:

1. Rub garlic clove on 1 side of each of the sourdough toasted bread slices
2. Spread sun dried tomatoes on garlic side of bread. Drizzle in olive oil and sprinkle chives.
3. Pop bread into the oven toaster. Transfer to a plate. Serve warm.

Cheesy Strawberry Sandwich

Ingredients:
- 1 slice rye bread
- 1 tsp. strawberry jam or any jam of choice
- 1 tsp. gouda cheese, shredded
- 1 tsp. cottage cheese
- ½ tsp. butter, for frying

Directions:
1. Spread jam on 1 side of the rye bread. Slice in half.
2. Combine Gouda cheese and cottage cheese on 1 bread slice. Top off with the other slice.
3. Meanwhile, put just the right amount of butter on a skillet. Toast sandwich for 3 minutes on both sides.
4. Serve with fresh berries.

Coconut and Buttery Yam

Ingredients:

- 1 yam, unpeeled
- water, for boiling
- Pinch of sea salt, add more if needed
- 1 tsp. coconut butter, sugar-free
- 1 tsp. green stevia
- 1½ tsp. desiccated coconut, toasted

Directions:

1. Put yam in a saucepan. Pour just enough water to submerge yam. Season with salt. Put the lid on and bring to a boil.
2. Reduce the heat and allow to simmer for 30 minutes.
3. Turn off the heat. Remove yam from the saucepan. Rinse under running water. Drain.
4. Once cool enough to handle, peel yam. Place peeled yam in a bowl and add coconut butter. Mash using a potato masher. Divide into 4 equal portions.
5. Using an ice cream scooper, ladle out equal portions on a plate. Create a small well in the center.

6. Put together stevia and desiccated coconut. Sprinkle on top of the mashed yam. Serve.

Garlic Bread with Two Cheeses

Ingredients:

- 1 garlic clove, minced
- 1 tsp. butter
- ½ tsp. fresh parsley, minced
- 1 sugar-free sourdough roll
- 1 Tbsp. parmesan cheese, grated
- 1 tsp. Asiago cheese
- 1 slice German ham, julienned

Directions:

1. Combine garlic, butter, and parsley in a bowl. Spread on bread. Top with ham pieces into bread.
2. Sprinkle shaved parmesan and Asiago cheese.
3. Heat the bread in the oven toaster. Serve warm.

Avocado and Pumpkin Seed Parfait

Ingredients:

- 1 tablespoon cashew nuts, chopped

For the Parfait Base

- 1 banana, mashed
- 2 tablespoons pumpkin seeds
- ⅛ teaspoon nutmeg powder
- ½ teaspoon cinnamon powder
- 1¼ cups almond milk

For the Avocado Jam

- 2 avocados, diced
- 2 tablespoons chia seeds
- ⅛ teaspoon nutmeg powder
- ¾ teaspoon cinnamon powder
- Pinch of sea salt

Directions:

1. Combine banana, pumpkin seeds, almond milk, nutmeg powder, cinnamon powder in a bowl, Mix until well combined. Chill in the fridge.

2. Meanwhile, in a saucepan set over medium heat. Combine avocados, nutmeg powder, cinnamon powder, and salt. Bring to a boil. Allow to simmer for 20 minutes.

3. Turn off the heat. Mash half of the jam using a wooden spoon. Let cool. Set aside.

4. Spoon 2 tablespoons of parfait base and apple jam into parfait glasses. Garnish with cashew nuts. Serve.

Chicken and Macaroni Fruit Cocktail Salad

Ingredients:

- ¼ cup macaroni salad, cooked
- ¼ cup boiled chicken, diced into bite-sized pieces
- ¼ cup fruit cocktail, syrup drained well
- 2 Tbsp. mayonnaise, low-fat
- 1 Tbsp. sour cream
- 1 Tbsp. cottage cheese
- 1 tsp. raisins
- 1 tsp. celery, minced
- Pinch of sea salt, add more if needed
- Pinch of black pepper, to taste

Directions:

1. Whisk mayonnaise, sour cream, and cottage cheese until creamy.
2. Fold in remaining ingredients. Season well with salt and pepper. Chill for 1 hour before serving. This will make the raisins plump up too.
3. Divide into 2 equal portions. Serve plain or with sugar-free bread/saltines.

Crostini with Salmon

Ingredients:

- 2 slices wheat bread, toasted
- 2 garlic cloves, peeled
- 4 smoked salmon slivers
- 2 sprigs fresh chives, minced
- 1 tablespoon capers
- ¼ cup tomatoes, minced
- ½ cup cucumbers, minced
- Pinch of sea salt
- Pinch of white pepper
- 2 tablespoon lemon juice, freshly squeezed

Directions:

1. Preheat the oven toaster. Rub garlic cloves on the toasted bread. Set aside.
2. In a small bowl, combine salmon, capers, tomatoes, cucumbers, salt, and pepper. Adjust seasoning.
3. Spread on bread slices. Place in the oven toaster to warm through. Garnish with chives and sprinkle lemon juice. Serve.

Spinach and Bacon Crostini

Ingredients:
- 2 slices wheat bread, toasted
- 2 garlic cloves, peeled

For the Toppings:
- 2 tablespoons water
- 4 streaky bacon
- 1 teaspoon Dijon mustard
- 1 teaspoon apple cider vinegar
- 1 handful baby-spinach leaves
- 1 handful arugula leaves
- Pinch of sea salt
- Pinch of white pepper

Directions:
1. Rub garlic cloves on the toasted bread. Set aside.
2. In a skillet set over high heat, pour water and layer the bacon. Cook until crisp. Place bacon on the bread.
3. Whisk Dijon mustard and apple cider vinegar into the bacon fat. Stir until the dressing

blends and emulsifies. Tip in spinach and arugula leaves. Season with salt and pepper.

4. Add equal portions on top of bacon slices. Serve.

Nectarine White Tea Cold Brew

Ingredients:
- 4 cups water
- 4 teabags white tea
- 1 apple, diced into bite-sized pieces
- 1 nectarine, diced into bite-sized pieces

Directions:
1. Combine all ingredients into large non-reactive pitcher or container. Place lid on.
2. Steep tea in fridge for 5 hours. Strain out and discard spent teabags.
3. Divide brew into 2 equal portions. Serve with apple and nectarine pieces.

Pecan-Almond Butter

Ingredients:

- ¾ cup raw pecans, chopped
- 1 cup raw blanched almond slivers
- 1 vanilla pod, halved lengthwise
- ¼ teaspoon sea salt

Directions:

1. Preheat the oven to 350°F.
2. Line a baking sheet with aluminum foil. Spread nuts on the baking sheet. Bake for 10 minutes or until golden brown.
3. Remove from heat. Cool before placing into food processor. Add vanilla pod, honey, and salt. Process until smooth. Store in airtight container.

Dried Apple and White Tea

- freshly boiled water for making tea

Oven-Dried Apples
- 2 apples, thinly sliced
- 2 Tbsp. lemon juice, freshly-squeezed
- 2 Tbsp. coconut sugar
- 1 cup ice cubes
- filtered water for soaking

For the tea
- 15 whole cloves
- 1 cinnamon stick, crumbled
- ½ cup loose-leaf white tea

Directions:
1. Preheat oven to 200°F. Line two baking sheets with parchment paper. Set aside.
2. After slicing apples, quickly place these along with lemon juice and ice cubes in a large bowl. Pour enough water to completely submerge apples under an inch of liquid. Soak for 5 minutes.

3. Drain apples, and then pat dry using tea towels.

4. Arrange apple slices on prepared baking sheets, making sure none overlap.

5. Lightly sprinkle with coconut sugar.

6. Bake apples for 90 minutes. If apples are browning too fast, turn off heat immediately, but leave the apples in the oven to dry in the residual heat. Remove baking sheets from oven.

7. Let apples cool completely to room temperature before mincing.

8. For the tea, combine half of dried minced apples with tea ingredients. Mix well. Store in airtight container until ready to use. This recipe is good for multiple servings.

9. Take 1 heaping tablespoon of tea mix and place into tea pot. Fill with desired amount of freshly-boiled water. Steep for 5 to 7 minutes.

10. Strain tea into cups. Serve with more dried apples on the side.

Conclusion

Thank you again for purchasing this book!

I hope this book was able to help you know more about the South Beach Diet and the kind of food that you should eat, limit, and completely avoid. The recipes found here will also help you get started with the diet program, one day at a time. All the recipes that are found in this cookbook will help you live a healthy and improved lifestyle.

The next step is to try out the recipes and create some variations provided that you follow Phases 1, 2, and 3 recipes to the letter.

Once again, don't forget to grab a copy of your FREE BONUS book "Super Foods For Super Health". If you are interested in learning more about the easily accessible super foods that you could incorporate into your diet and transform your overall health, then this book is for you.

Just go to http://bit.ly/superfoods-gift

Thank you and good luck!

Thank you!

Before you go, I just wanted to say thank you for purchasing my book.

You could have picked from dozens of other books on the same topic but you took a chance and chose this one.

So, a HUGE thanks to you for getting this book and for reading all the way to the end.

Now I wanted to ask you for a small favor. **Could you please take just a few minutes to leave a review for this book on Amazon?**

This feedback will help me continue to write the type of books that will help you get the results you want. So if you enjoyed it, please let me know! (-:

79290728R00092

Made in the USA
Lexington, KY
20 January 2018